TREAT YOUR OWN

NECK

ROBIN McKENZIE

SPINAL PUBLICATIONS NEW ZEALAND LTD

Treat Your Own Neck

First Edition, first published in 1983
Second Revised Edition August, 2006

Spinal Publications New Zealand Ltd
1 Alexander Road, PO Box 2026
Raumati Beach, New Zealand
Email: enquiries@spinalpublications.co.nz
Telephone: ++ 64 4 299-7020

ISBN-13   978-0-9582692-1-6
ISBN-10   0-9582692-1-1

Designed and typeset by Astra Print
Edited by Autumnwood Editing
Photography by John Cheese
Printed and bound by Astra Print

Acknowledgements

I would like to thank senior faculty members Hugh Murray (USA), Robert Medcalf (USA) and Colin Davies (Canada) of the McKenzie Institute International for the many helpful suggestions they have provided for the content of this second revision of *Treat Your Own Neck*.

I would also like to acknowledge the work done by my daughter, Jan McKenzie, and Jenny Bertelsen (manager of Spinal Publications New Zealand Ltd) in revising the layout and format and for their persistence without which I would still be months behind the deadline.

Finally, many thanks to Niniwa Roberts and Treena Fitness for modelling the exercises over the years.

Robin McKenzie

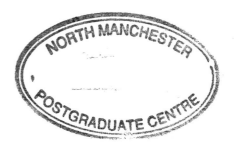

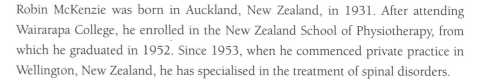

About the author

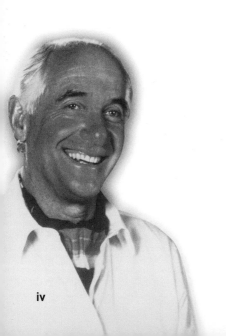

Robin McKenzie was born in Auckland, New Zealand, in 1931. After attending Wairarapa College, he enrolled in the New Zealand School of Physiotherapy, from which he graduated in 1952. Since 1953, when he commenced private practice in Wellington, New Zealand, he has specialised in the treatment of spinal disorders.

During the 1960s Robin McKenzie developed his own examination and treatment methods and is now recognised internationally as an authority on the diagnosis and treatment of low back and neck pain. He has lectured internationally and, to give some indication of the success of the system of treatment he has developed, the McKenzie Method of mechanical diagnosis and therapy (MDT) is now taught and practised worldwide. In the United States, the United Kingdom, Ireland and in New Zealand, the McKenzie Method is the preferred treatment of choice among physiotherapists for back problems.

In June 2004, the journal *ADVANCE* for Physical Therapists and PT Assistants (USA) published the results of a survey sent to a random sampling of 320 physical therapists from the orthopaedic section of the American Physical Therapy Association. The therapists were asked which physical therapists or physicians of all time had the strongest influence on their thinking or performance in orthopaedic physical therapy. The clinicians voted the number one most influential was Robin McKenzie.

The success of the McKenzie Method has attracted intense interest from researchers in various parts of the world, and it is one of the most studied diagnostic and treatment systems for back and neck pain at the present time. An extensive list of scientific studies carried out worldwide demonstrates the efficacy and importance of the diagnostic process and the treatment system. If you are interested in reading more about this, visit the website www.mckenziemdt.org.

To ensure the orderly development of education and research into the methods devised by Robin McKenzie, doctors and physiotherapists involved in the teaching process formed the McKenzie Institute International in 1982. The Institute is a not-for-profit organisation with headquarters in New Zealand. Robin McKenzie was elected the first president of the Institute.

Robin McKenzie has published in *The New Zealand Medical Journal* and contributed to many authoritative texts on back and neck problems. He is the author of six books: *Treat Your Own Back* (1980), *Treat Your Own Neck* (1983), *Seven Steps to a Pain Free Life* (2000), *The Lumbar Spine: Mechanical Diagnosis & Therapy* (1981 and 2003), *The Cervical & Thoracic Spine: Mechanical Diagnosis & Therapy* (1990 and 2006) and *The Human Extremities: Mechanical Diagnosis & Therapy* (2000).

The contributions Robin McKenzie has made to the understanding and treatment of musculoskeletal problems have been internationally recognised. In 1982 he was made an Honorary Life Member of the American Physical Therapy Association "in recognition of distinguished and meritorious service to the art and science of physical therapy and to the welfare of mankind."

In 1983 he was elected to membership of the International Society for the Study of the Lumbar Spine. In 1984 he was made a Fellow of the American Back Society, and in 1985 he was awarded an Honorary Fellowship of the New Zealand Society of Physiotherapists. In 1987 he was made an Honorary Life Member of the New Zealand Manipulative Therapists Association and in 1990 an Honorary Fellow of the Chartered Society of Physiotherapists in the United Kingdom.

In the 1990 Queen's Birthday Honours, he was made an Officer of the Most Excellent Order of the British Empire (OBE). In the New Year Honours 2000, Her Majesty Queen Elizabeth II appointed Robin McKenzie to be a Companion of the New Zealand Order of Merit (CNZM).

Contents

x

Neck problems

Neck problems are referred to in different ways such as arthritis in the neck, spondylosis of the neck, rheumatism, fibrositis, slipped disc or, when it concerns pain extending into the arm, neuritis and neuralgia.

At some time during our lives, most of us suffer from pain in the region of the neck, or pain arising from the neck that is felt across the shoulders, in the shoulder blade or the upper or lower arm. Pain coming from the neck can also be felt in the hand, and symptoms such as pins and needles or numbness can be experienced in the fingers. Some people are troubled by headaches, the cause of which can be traced to problems in the neck.

Usually these aches and pains occur intermittently – that is, there are days or times in the day that no pain is felt. The symptoms may appear mysteriously, often for no apparent reason, and just as mysteriously they disappear. These aches and pains may also occur constantly – that is, pain to some degree is felt at all times. People who have pain all of the time are frequently forced to take medication and sometimes have to stop work. The pain simply makes their lives miserable and they have to reduce their activities in order to keep the discomfort at a moderate level. Neck problems can thus affect our lifestyle.

If you have problems of this nature, you may already have discovered that the symptoms can sometimes last for months or even years. You may have found that treatments are often able to stop your pain, but the pain returns later to affect you once more. You may be reading this book because you have persistent pains that have not disappeared, despite the fact that you may have received many types of treatments. Whatever the situation, you most likely realise that many of the treatments dispensed by doctors, physiotherapists and chiropractors are prescribed for your present symptoms and are not directed at preventing future problems. Time and again you may have to seek assistance to get relief from your neck pain. How good would it be if you were able to apply treatment to yourself whenever pain arose? Better still, how good would it be if you were able to apply a system of treatment to yourself that would prevent the onset of pain?

It has been shown repeatedly that patients require a rational explanation for their problems. They need education in postures and exercises that allow them to remain free of disabling symptoms. They need advice on how to avoid the detrimental forces encountered in daily living and how to apply beneficial strategies. All of these things are found in this book.

Since the 1970s, methods have been discovered that enable us to learn to manage our own spinal problems. The self-treatment methods I am going to describe to you evolved after my experiences with more than 20,000 patients during forty years of practice. The methods have been used by doctors and physiotherapists in many parts of the world for decades, and generally their patients are achieving the same satisfactory results.

Radiographic studies[1] in the United States have confirmed that the exercises described in this book restore the neck posture to its proper anatomical alignment. Another study[2] validating the efficacy of these exercises in patients with arm and neck pain showed a reduction in symptoms and improvement in reflex activity. When the neck was held in a forward bent position, the pain increased and reflexes worsened.

One of the main points of this book is that the management of your neck is your responsibility. If, for some reason or other, you have developed neck problems, then you must learn how to deal with the present symptoms and how to prevent future problems. Self-treatment will be more effective in the long term management of your neck pain than any other form of treatment.

[1] Ordway NR, Seymour RJ, Donelson RG, Hojnowski LS, Edwards WT (1999). Cervical flexion, extension, protrusion, and retraction: A radiographic segmental analysis. Spine 24 (3).240-7.

[2] Abdulwahab SS, Sabbahi M (2000) Neck retractions, cervical root decompression, and radicular pain. J Orthop Sports Phys Ther. 30 (1).4-9.

Who can perform self-treatment?

This book is meant for those with straightforward *recurring* mechanical problems. There are only a few people who will not benefit from the advice given in this book. Nearly everyone can commence the exercise programme, provided the recommended precautions are taken.

Once you have started the exercises, carefully watch your pain pattern. If your pains are getting progressively worse and remain worse the following day, or if they are slowly increasing in severity and becoming intolerable, you should seek advice from your doctor or a McKenzie Institute International credentialled or diplomaed clinician.

If you have developed neck or shoulder pain for the *first* time you should consult your doctor who will perhaps refer you to a physiotherapist for treatment and, more importantly, for advice and instructions on the prevention of further neck problems. You should also seek advice if there are complications to your neck problems, for example if you have severe and stabbing pains, if your head is pulled off-centre or if you have severe persisting headaches.

In any of the following situations you should *not* commence the exercise programme without first consulting your doctor or physiotherapist:

- if you have pain near or at the wrist or hand and experience sensations of pins and needles or numbness in the fingers
- if you have developed neck problems following a recent, severe accident

- if you have developed headaches recently; in this case your eyes or prescription glasses may need to be checked
- if you experience severe headaches that have come on for no apparent reason, never cease and are gradually getting worse
- if you have severe episodic headaches that are accompanied by nausea and dizziness.

Choose your therapist carefully. You should be provided with the information and education you require to manage your own problem. Every patient deserves to have the opportunity to learn how to manage their own neck pain, and every therapist should be obligated to provide that information.

The only health care professionals fully qualified to provide the McKenzie Method are members of the McKenzie Institute International who hold the credentialling certificate or the Diploma in Mechanical Diagnosis & Therapy®. To obtain names of treatment providers trained by the McKenzie Institute, see the directory at the back of this book or use the search feature on the McKenzie Institute International website: www.mckenziemdt.org.

This book describes a complete system of management, which must be followed in its *entirety* to ensure success.

Do *not* turn straight to the exercise description pages; your understanding of the preceding chapters is *essential*.

Vertebrae and the spine

Let us look at the human backbone, the spine or spinal column (Photo 1). In the neck area the spine consists of seven bones, the vertebrae, which rest upon one another similar to a stack of cotton spools (Photo 2).

Each vertebra has a solid part in front, called the vertebral body, and a hole in the back. When lined up as the spinal column these holes form the spinal canal (Photo 3). This canal serves as a protected passageway for the spinal cord, the bundle of nerves that extends from head to pelvis.

Separating the vertebrae are special cartilages, called the discs. These are located between the vertebral bodies just in front of the spinal cord (Photo 2). Each disc consists of a soft fluid centre, the nucleus, which is surrounded and held together by a cartilage ring – the annulus or annular ligament. The discs are similar to rubber washers and act as shock absorbers. They are able to alter their shape, thus allowing movement of one vertebra on another and of the neck as a whole.

The vertebrae and discs are linked up by a series of joints to form the cervical spine or neck. Each joint is held together by its surrounding soft tissues – that is, a capsule reinforced by ligaments. Muscles lie over one or more joints of the neck and may

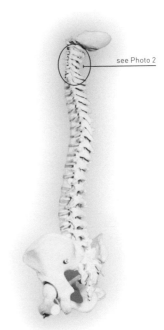

see Photo 2

Photo 1
The spine or spinal column

7

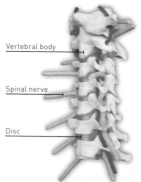

Vertebral body

Spinal nerve

Disc

Photo 2
Seven cervical vertebrae with discs
between and nerve roots showing

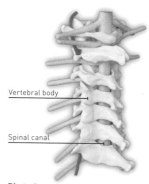

Vertebral body

Spinal canal

Photo 3
Cervical vertebrae viewed from the
back, showing the holes that form
the spinal canal

extend upwards to the head or downwards to the trunk. At both ends each muscle changes into a tendon by which it attaches itself to different bones. When a muscle contracts it causes movement in one or more joints.

Between each two vertebrae there is a small opening on either side through which a nerve leaves the spinal canal – the right and left spinal nerve (Photo 2). Among other tasks the spinal nerves supply our muscles with power and our skin with sensation. The nerves are really part of our alarm system: pain is the warning that some structure is about to be damaged or has already sustained some damage.

Research has shown that the disc consists of tough cartilage material that early in life develops splits (called fissures). These fissures allow fragments of loose material within the disc to displace to the back of the joint where they may become trapped and cause pain.

Functions of the cervical spine

On top of this complex of bones and washers rests the head, which contains our computer system, the brain, and the important sensors associated with it such as the eyes, ears, nose and mouth. Together, the vertebrae, discs and head form a series of flexible joints that allow the head to turn almost 180 degrees from one side to the other, to look up and down, and to bend sideways. In addition, the head can adopt many positions that are combinations of these movements.

The main functions of the cervical spine are to support the head, allow it to move in many directions and adjust its position in fine degrees in order to assist the working of the sensors and to provide a protected passageway for the bundle of nerves that extends from the brain to the sacrum, the tail end of the spine.

The neck has a high flexibility due to the specially designed structure of the joints, in particular those between the uppermost vertebrae and the head. Its flexibility is further increased because no bony structures are attached to the spine in this area. Thus, the neck can move relatively more freely than the rest of the spine where movements are restricted by the ribcage and pelvis. On the other hand, because the neck is not surrounded and protected by other structures, it is also more vulnerable than the rest of the spine when subjected to strains. Its very flexibility, so helpful and necessary for everyday living, is also the cause of many of our problems. The wide range of movement of the neck exposes it to an equally wide range of stresses and strains.

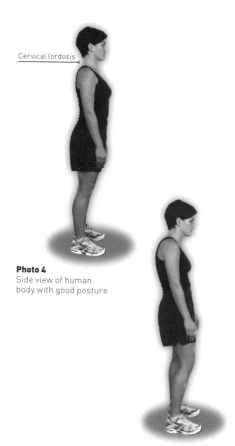

Cervical lordosis

Photo 4
Side view of human
body with good posture

Photo 5
Bad posture

Natural posture

The side view of the human body (Photo 4) shows that there is a small inward curve in the neck just above the shoulder girdle. This is called the cervical lordosis. It is this curve in the spine that mainly concerns us in this book.

When standing upright the head should be carried directly above the shoulder girdle, thus forming a small but visible cervical lordosis (Photo 4). Due to postural neglect people can often be seen to carry the head in front of their body with their chin poking forward (Photo 5). Now the cervical lordosis is altered in shape and distorted. In this position the joints of the lower neck are relatively bent forwards or flexed, whereas those between the upper part of the neck and the head are bent backwards or extended. This is called the protruded head posture (Photo 5). If present often and long enough, neck problems may develop.

Mechanical pain

Pain of mechanical origin occurs when the joint between two bones has been placed in a position that overstretches the surrounding ligaments and other soft tissues. This is true for mechanical pain in any joint of the body, including the spine. To help you understand how easily some mechanical pains can be produced, you may like to try a simple experiment.

First, bend one finger backward until you feel a strain, as shown in Photo 6. If you keep your finger in this position, you initially feel only minor discomfort, but as time passes, pain eventually develops. In some cases, pain caused by prolonged stretching may take as much as an hour to appear.

Try the experiment once more, but now keep bending the finger past the point of strain until you feel the immediate sensation of pain. You have overstretched, and your pain warning system is telling you that to continue movement in that particular direction will cause damage.

The pain warning tells you to stop overstretching to avoid damage and, when you do so, the pain ceases immediately. No damage has occurred and the pain has gone. No lasting problems arise from this short-lived strain providing you take note of the pain warning system.

If you fail to heed the warning and keep the finger in the overstretched position, the ligaments and surrounding soft tissues that hold the joint together will eventually tear. This tearing will result in an ache that continues even when you stop overstretching. The pain reduces in intensity but continues even when the finger is at rest. The pain increases with movement performed in the wrong direction and will not cease until some healing has occurred. Healing may take several days, but would be prolonged if every day you were to continue to apply the same strains to the finger. The same things happen when you overstretch the ligaments in your neck.

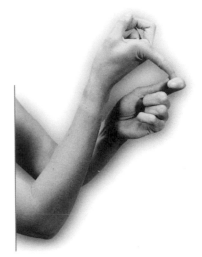

Photo 6
Bend the finger until you feel the strain

Mechanical neck pain

In the spine, the tissues that surround the joints between the vertebrae (in particular the ligaments) are also responsible for supporting the soft discs that separate the vertebrae. They hold the discs in an enclosed compartment and help to form a shock absorbing mechanism. Mechanical neck pain may arise due to *overstretching* these tissues.

Overstretching

The ligaments and other soft tissues that hold the vertebrae together can simply be overstretched without further damage. Overstretching may be caused by an outside force placing a sudden severe strain on the neck, for example due to an accident or during contact sport. This type of stress cannot easily be avoided as it occurs unexpectedly. More often overstretching is caused by postural stresses that place less severe strains on the neck over a longer time period. This type of stress is exerted by us on our own necks and can easily be influenced. Here lies our main responsibility in the self-treatment and prevention of neck pain.

Tissue damage

Complications arise when overstretching of soft tissues leads to actual *tissue damage*.

It is often thought that neck pain is caused by strained muscles. This is not the case. Muscles, which are the source of power and cause movement, can be overstretched but usually heal rapidly and seldom cause pain lasting for more than a week or two. However, underlying soft tissues that provide support for spinal joints such as capsules and ligaments are readily injured from overstretching. In fact, usually these are damaged long before the muscles. Thus, the real problem lies in and about the affected joint. When these soft tissues heal they may form scar tissues, become less elastic and shorten. At this stage even normal movements may stretch the scars in these shortened structures and produce pain. Unless appropriate exercises are performed to gradually stretch and lengthen these structures and restore their normal flexibility, they may become a continuous source of neck pain or headaches.

Bulging disc

Complications of another nature arise when the ligaments surrounding the disc are injured to such an extent that the disc loses its ability to absorb shock and its outer wall becomes weakened. This allows the soft inside of the disc to bulge outwards and, in extreme cases, to burst through the outer ligament, which may cause serious problems. When the disc bulge protrudes far enough backwards it may press painfully on a spinal nerve. This may cause some of the pains felt well away from the source of the trouble, for example in the arm or hand.

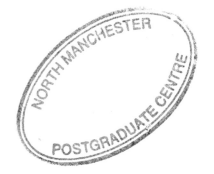

Due to this bulging the disc may become severely distorted and prevent the vertebrae from lining up properly during movement. In this case some movements may be blocked partially or completely and forcing of these movements causes severe pain. This is the reason that in some people the head can only be held in an off-centre position. Those of you who experience a sudden onset of pain and following this are unable to move the head normally may have some bulging of the soft disc material. This need not be a cause for alarm. The movements described in this book are carefully designed to reduce any disturbance of this nature.

Pain location

The sites of pain caused by neck problems vary from one person to another:

In a **first attack**, pain is usually felt:

- at or near the base of the neck, in the centre (Figure 1), *or*
- just to one side (Figure 2).

Usually these pains subside within a few days.

In **subsequent attacks** pain may:

- reach across both shoulders (Figure 3)
- to the top of one shoulder or the shoulder blade (Figure 4), *and*
- later still to the outside or back of the upper arm as far as the elbow (Figure 5), *or*
- it may extend below the elbow to the wrist or hand, and pins and needles or numbness may be felt in the fingers (Figure 6)

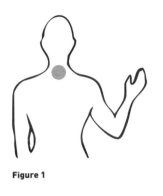

Figure 1

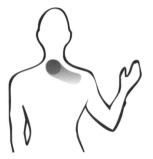

Figure 2

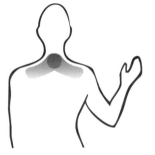

Figure 3

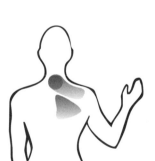

Figure 4

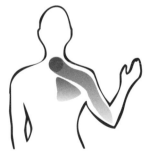

Figure 5

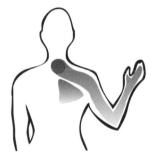

Figure 6

Some people experience **headaches** as a result of neck problems. Often headaches are felt:

- at the top of the neck and the base and the back of the head, on one or both sides (Figure 7)
- extending from the base of the back of the head to just below the crown of the head (Figure 8 – *occipital headache*)
- spreading from the back of the head over the top of the head to above or behind the eye, again on one or both sides (Figure 9 – *total headache*)
- distributed across the forehead and often felt behind the eyes (Figure 10 – *frontal headache*)
- distributed around the head, often described as feeling like a "tight band" (Figure 11 – *circumferential headache*).

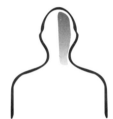

Figure 7

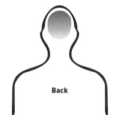

Back

Figure 8

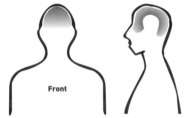

Front

Figure 9

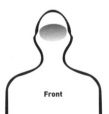

Front

Figure 10

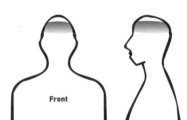

Front

Figure 11

Postural stresses

The most common form of neck pain is caused by overstretching of ligaments due to postural stresses. This may occur when sitting with poor posture for a long time (Photo 7), when lying or sleeping with the head in an awkward position (Photos 8 and 9) and when working in strained positions (Photo 10). When you look carefully at these photos, you will see that the cervical lordosis is no longer present.

Of all these postural stresses, the poor sitting posture – that is, sitting with the head protruded – is by far the one most often at fault. Poor posture in itself may produce neck pain. Once neck problems have developed however, poor posture will frequently make them worse and always perpetuate them.

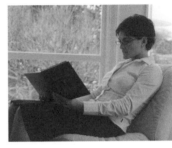

Photo 7
Bad sitting position

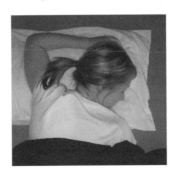

Photo 8
Bad sleeping posture

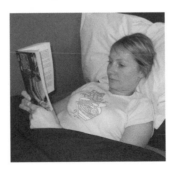

Photo 9
Bad lying posture

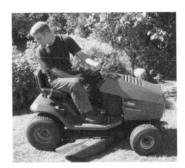

Photo 10
Strained working position

The main theme of this chapter is that pain of postural origin will not occur if you avoid prolonged overstretching. Should pain develop, there are certain movements you can perform in order to stop that pain. You should *not* have to seek assistance whenever postural pain arises.

Consequences of postural neglect

Unfortunately many of us spend much of our work and leisure time with the neck in a protruded position and lose the lordosis completely. On the other hand, we seldom or never increase it to its maximum. If you reduce the lordosis for long periods at a time and never properly restore it, you eventually lose the ability to form the hollow.

Some people who habitually adopt poor postures and remain unaware of the underlying cause experience neck pain throughout their lifetimes simply because they were not in possession of the necessary information to correct the postural faults.

When pains of postural origin are first felt they are easily eliminated merely by correcting the posture. However, as time passes, the uncorrected habitual poor posture causes changes to the structure and shape of the joints; excessive wear occurs, with loss of elasticity resulting in premature ageing of the joints. The effects of poor posture in the long term therefore, can be just as severe and harmful as the effects of injury.

Sitting for prolonged periods

When we are moving about, especially when walking briskly, we assume a fairly upright posture. The head is retracted and held directly over the vertebral column and consequently receives the maximum support possible. When we sit and relax in a chair (Photo 11), the head and neck slowly protrude because the muscles that support them become tired. As the muscles tire they relax, and so we lose the main support for a good posture. The result is the protruded head posture (Photo 12). This posture can be seen around us every day. It is not present during infancy, but develops from mid-teens onwards. We are not really designed to sit for six to eight hours daily, up to six days a week.

When the protruded head posture is maintained long enough, it causes overstretching of ligaments. Thus pain will arise only in certain positions. Once the protruded posture has become a habit and is maintained most of the time, it may also cause distortion of the discs contained in the vertebral joints. At this stage, movements as well as positions will produce pain. Neck problems developed in this way are the consequence of postural neglect. Poor neck posture is not the only cause of neck pain. It is, however, one of the main causes and the most troublesome perpetuating factor.

During sitting, the position of the low back strongly influences the posture of the neck. If the low back is allowed to slouch, it is impossible to sit with head and neck pulled backwards. You can easily try this out for yourself. Unfortunately, once we have been sitting in a certain position for a few minutes, our body sags and we end

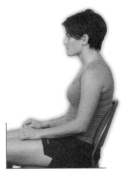

Photo 11
Bad sitting posture

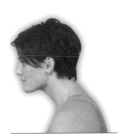

Photo 12
Protruded head posture

21

up sitting slouched with a rounded low back and protruded head and neck. For most people, sitting for prolonged periods results in poor posture.

Environmental factors

The design of transportation, commercial and domestic seating only encourages our poor postural habits. Although most seats nowadays have some level of lumbar support, rarely do the chairs available give adequate support to the low back and neck and, unless a conscious effort is made to sit correctly, we are forced to sit badly. For the neck, ideally the back of the chair should come up high enough so that we can rest our head against it, but this support is not always included. An exception is the seating manufactured for most airlines but, unfortunately, their head-supports generally push the head and neck into the protruded position which causes our problems. When travelling by car, train, bus or plane we are often compelled to sit in the position dictated by the seats provided. It may be necessary for the driver of a car, bus or truck, especially in bad weather, to protrude head and neck in order to peer through the windscreen.

Domestic furniture has not received the same design improvements that have been made in the office and commercial field. Unless your favourite lounge-chair is exceptional, you will have insufficient support for the low back and neck, and you will continue to place strains on these areas when you relax for the evening. If your neck problems are aggravated by reading or watching television, it is unlikely that the content of the book, newspaper or television programme is giving you the pain in the neck; the posture that you have adopted is the cause of the pain, and this posture depends to a large extent on the type of chair or support you use.

Although the poor design of furniture contributes to the development of neck problems, equal blame lies with the way in which we use this furniture. If we do not know how to sit correctly, even the best designed chairs will not prevent us from slouching. On the other hand, once we are educated in correct sitting, bad chairs need not have a big impact on our posture.

How to manage prolonged sitting situations

In order to prevent the development of neck pain due to prolonged poor sitting, it is necessary to:

1. sit correctly, and
2. interrupt the protruded head posture or prolonged neck bending at regular intervals.

In order to treat neck pain resulting from poor posture, other exercises may need to be performed besides the postural correction. In this chapter I only discuss the exercises required to reduce postural stresses and obtain postural correction. The exercises for relief of pain and increase of function will be dealt with in Chapters 5 and 6.

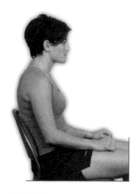

Photo 13
Poor neck posture: the result of
insufficient low back support

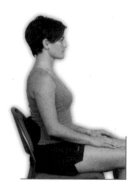

Photo 14
Good neck posture made possible
with low back support

Correction of the sitting posture

You may have been sitting slouched for many years without neck and shoulder pain. However, once you have developed neck problems you must no longer sit in the old way, because this posture will only perpetuate the overstretching discussed previously.

If you are sitting slouched with the low back rounded, it is not possible to correct the posture of the neck (Photo 13). Therefore it is necessary to first correct the posture of your low back. How to assume and maintain the correct posture of the low back in sitting is described in my other book, *Treat Your Own Back*. However, for the purposes of this book, you must be fully aware of the following.

To sit correctly (Photo 14), you must *maintain* the natural hollow (lordosis) that is present in your low back while standing. To maintain your lordosis it is helpful to use a lumbar roll. This is a specially designed support for your low back (Photos 15 and 16). The roll should be made of foam and be no more than five to six inches in diameter before being compressed. Without this support your low back slouches and your head protrudes as soon as you relax or concentrate on anything other than your posture; for example, when talking, reading, writing, working behind a computer, watching television or driving the car.

To counteract this slouching, place a lumbar roll in the small of your back, about the level of your beltline, whenever you sit in an easy chair, car or office chair (Photos 17-22).

The Original McKenzie® range of lumbar rolls is available worldwide from a supplier, listed at the back of this book. Proceeds from the sale of the Original McKenzie® spinal supports have been, and continue to be, donated for research into improved methods of treatment for musculoskeletal disorders and to provide relevant education for health care professionals.

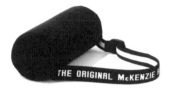

Photo 15
The Original McKenzie®
Regular Lumbar Roll

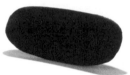

Photo 16
The Original McKenzie®
SuperRoll

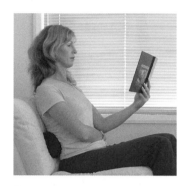

Photo 17
Correct

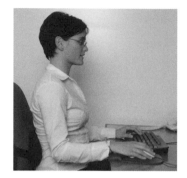

Photo 19
Correct

Photo 21
Correct

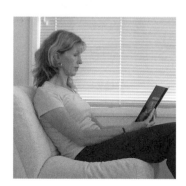

Photo 18
Incorrect

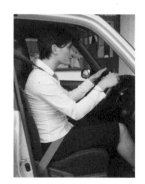

Photo 20
Incorrect

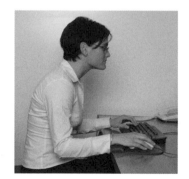

Photo 22
Incorrect

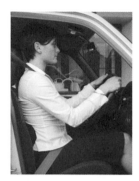

In order to correct the posture of your neck while sitting, you must first learn how to retract the head. Therefore you must become fully practised in *Exercise 1: Head retraction in sitting* (see Chapter 5, page 42). This exercise should be performed 15 to 20 times per session and the session should be repeated three times per day, preferably morning, noon and evening. This rhythmic procedure teaches you the correct position of your head in relation to the rest of your body. Each backward movement of the head must be performed to the maximum possible degree. When the head is pulled back as far as possible, you have assumed the so-called *retracted head posture* (Photo 23).

Now you have reached the extreme of the corrected head and neck posture.

Correct head posture

Once you know how to retract the head, you must learn how to find and maintain the correct head and neck posture. The extreme of the retracted head position is a position of strain and it is not possible to sit in this way for a long time. To sit comfortably and correctly you must hold your head just short of the extreme retracted posture. To find this position you must first retract the head as far as possible (Photo 23) and then release the last ten percent of this movement (Photo 24). Now you have reached the correct head and neck posture, which can be maintained for any length of time. It may take up to eight days of practise to master this.

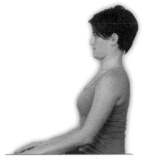

Photo 23
Retracted head posture

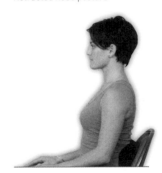

Photo 24
Correct head posture

When sitting for prolonged periods you must sit correctly, with the low back supported by a lumbar roll and the head slightly retracted.

The aim of this part of the programme is to first restore the correct posture and then maintain it. As a rule the pain decreases as your head posture improves and you will have no pain once you maintain the correct posture. The pain will readily recur in the first few weeks whenever you allow your head to protrude, but eventually you will remain completely pain-free even when you accidentally forget your posture. However, you should never again allow yourself to sit slouched with a protruded head for a long time. As soon as you have been completely pain-free for a couple of days, you can resume your normal activities. If from now on you follow the instructions given in this book, you may also be able to prevent further neck trouble.

When first commencing the above procedures to correct your low back and neck posture in sitting, you will experience some new pains. These may be different from your original pain and may be felt in another place. New pains are the result of performing new exercises and maintaining new positions. They should be expected and will wear off in a few days, provided postural correction is continued on a regular basis. Once you have become used to sitting correctly, you will enjoy it. You soon will notice the reduction or absence of pain and the increased comfort. From then on you will automatically choose chairs that allow you to sit correctly.

Regular interruption of prolonged neck bending

If you spend long periods of time in the sitting position (for example while knitting, reading or performing desk tasks) it is likely that, even with the best of intentions, you will eventually forget to maintain the correct posture. Gradually you will assume a more or less protruded head posture or a position in which both head and neck are bent forwards. To counteract this you must frequently interrupt the forward bent position by correcting your neck posture and stretching the head and neck backwards as described in *Exercise 2: Neck extension in sitting* (for full description see Chapter 5, page 44). This will relieve the stresses on the discs between the vertebrae as well as the surrounding tissues.

Lying and resting

The next most frequent cause of neck pain is postural stress in the lying position. If you wake up in the morning with a stiff and painful neck that was not causing problems the night before, there is likely to be something wrong with the surface on which you are lying or the position in which you sleep. It is a comparatively easy task to correct the surface on which you are lying, but rather difficult to influence the position you adopt while sleeping. Once you are asleep you may just regularly change your position or you may toss and turn. Unless a certain position causes so much discomfort that it wakes you up, you have no real idea of the various positions you assume while sleeping.

When sitting for prolonged periods, regular interruption of prolonged neck bending is essential. This can be achieved by retracting the head and extending the neck five or six times at regular intervals, for example each hour.

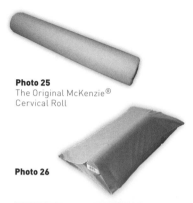

Photo 25
The Original McKenzie®
Cervical Roll

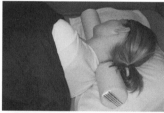

Photo 26

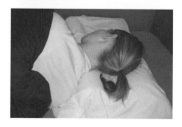

Photos 27 and 28

Correction of sleeping surface

All that is required to correct the surface on which you are lying is to alter your pillow. You may need to change the material of which it is made, the thickness of it, or both. You must realise that the main function of the pillow is to support both head and neck. Therefore it should fill the natural hollow in the contour of the neck between head and shoulder girdle without tilting the head or lifting it up. On the contrary, the head should be allowed to rest in a dish-shaped hollow, so you must be able to adjust the contents of the pillow easily. Normal pillows do not permit the head to rest into a dish-shaped hollow but tend to apply a recoil pressure against the natural position the head would like to adopt. If you have such a pillow, you should replace it with a feather/down pillow so you can easily adjust the contents to make a hollow for your head and bunch the edge to form a thick support for your neck.

Pillows made of moulded foam (including specially designed cervical pillows made of memory foam or tempura foam) do not allow their contents to be adjusted. They always adopt the shape of their original mould, irrespective of attempts to change them and this might not be suitable for your particular weight or shape.

If for some reason your pillow does not provide adequate support for your neck, you should also use a supportive roll. The Original McKenzie® Cervical Roll (Photo 25) is specifically designed for this purpose and, contrary to the 'static' cervical pillows, gives you the flexibility to alter its position to suit the shape of your cervical lordosis. This product is available worldwide from licensed suppliers (see back of this book).

Place the roll inside your pillowcase, on top of the pillow and along its lower edge (Photo 26). All neck supports need to fulfil individual requirements and each person needs to experiment for themselves for the most effective positioning (Photos 27 and 28).

Correction of the lying posture

If the lying posture itself is thought to cause the problems, it needs to be investigated for each person individually. There is one position which requires further discussion. Some people like to sleep lying face down and frequently wake up with a headache or pain in the neck, which wears off as the day progresses. Other than this they seem to have no neck problems.

While lying face down the head is usually turned to one side and in this position some of the joints, especially in the upper neck, reach the maximum possible degree of turning or may come very close to it (Photo 29). Consequently, this position places great strains on the soft tissues surrounding the joints of the neck and those between upper neck and head.

If you have problems of this nature, you must avoid lying face down. In addition, it is advisable that you perform the recommended exercises, in particular *Exercises 1, 2* and *6: Head retraction in sitting, Neck extension in sitting* and *Neck rotation* (see Chapter 5 for a full description). This is to ensure that you can retract the head, extend the neck properly and have an adequate range of movement when turning the head.

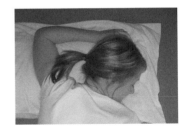

Photo 29
This sleeping position causes excessive strain

Relaxing after vigorous activity

When you have finished some vigorous activity for example, playing football, hockey, tennis, jogging or swimming – and have not suffered any pain as a result, you should not relax by sitting or lying with the head in the protruded posture (Photo 30). Thoroughly exercised joints of the spine easily distort if they are held in an overstretched position for prolonged periods. A common story is that a person sits down to rest following hard work, and some time later has such severe pain that the neck will hardly move. Usually the activity is blamed as the cause of the trouble, but in most cases the pain is produced by prolonged forward bending of head and neck when relaxing or resting afterwards.

Working in awkward positions or cramped spaces

Some jobs can only be performed in positions that are likely to cause overstretching of the neck. These jobs may require the adoption of the sitting position and usually they involve precision work. Alternatively, they may have to be performed in cramped spaces or with head and neck in awkward static positions (Photo 31). Under these circumstances you may not be able to prevent the onset of neck pain just by regularly assuming the correct posture. If your neck problems are brought on in this way you must, in addition to postural correction, frequently interrupt overstretching and perform *Exercise 6: Neck rotation*, and then *Exercises 1* and *2: Head retraction in sitting* and *Neck extension in sitting* (see Chapter 5 for a full description).

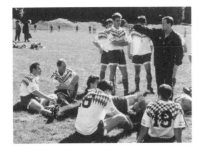

Photo 30
Relaxing after vigorous activity

After vigorous activity you should retract the head and extend the neck five or six times. If you sit down to rest, you should avoid the protruded head posture.

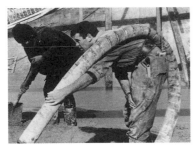

Photo 31
Awkward static working position

When working with the head and neck in a static position, you should at regular intervals interrupt this position by assuming the correct posture. In addition you should perform five or six movements of Exercise 6, and then Exercises 1 and 2.

Chapter four

YOUR UNDERSTANDING OF THIS CHAPTER IS ESSENTIAL FOR SUCCESSFUL SELF-TREATMENT. PLEASE READ IT CAREFULLY.

The aim of the exercises

The purpose of the exercises is to abolish pain and, where appropriate, to restore normal function – that is, to regain full mobility in the neck or as much movement as possible under the given circumstances.

When you are exercising for **pain relief**, you should move to the *edge of the pain* or *just into the pain*, then release the pressure and return to the starting position. When you are exercising for **stiffness**, the exercises can be made more effective by using your hands to gently but firmly and steadily apply *overpressure* in order to obtain the maximum amount of movement. Postural correction and maintenance of the correct posture should always follow the exercises. Once you no longer have neck pain, good postural habits are essential to prevent the recurrence of neck problems.

Effect on pain intensity and location

There are three main effects to look for while performing the exercises:

1. the exercise may cause the symptoms to disappear
2. they may cause an increase or decrease in the intensity of the pain that you experience

3. they may cause the pain to move from where you usually feel it to some other location.

In certain cases the symptoms first change locations, then they reduce in intensity and finally they cease altogether.

The effects of exercise on intensity or location of pain can sometimes be very rapid. It is possible to reduce the intensity or change the location of pain after completing as few as ten or twelve movements, and in some conditions the pain can completely disappear.

In order to determine whether the exercise programme is good for you, it is very important that you observe closely any changes in the location of the pain. You may notice that pain, originally felt to one side of the spine, across the shoulders or down the arm, moves towards the centre of your neck as a result of the exercises. In other words, your pain localises or *centralises*.

Centralisation

Centralisation is the movement of pain to a more central location, and centralisation of pain (Figure 12) that occurs as you exercise is a good sign. If your pain is usually felt further away from the neck and moves towards the midline of the cervical spine, you are exercising correctly and this exercise programme is the right one for you.

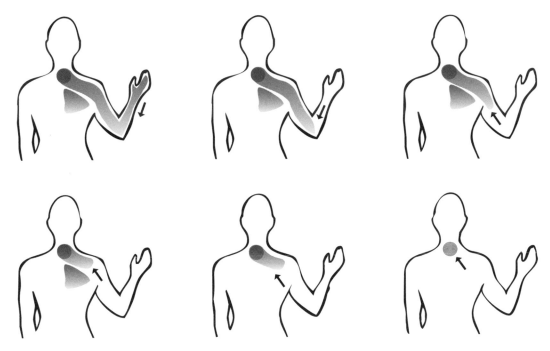

Figure 12
Progression of centralisation of pain indicates suitability of exercise programme

Pain intensity

If your neck pain is of such intensity that you can only move your head with difficulty and cannot find a position to lie comfortably in bed, your approach to the exercises should be cautious and unhurried.

On commencing any of the exercises you may experience an *increase* in pain. This initial pain increase is common and can be expected. As you continue to practise, the pain should quickly diminish, at least to its former level. Usually this occurs during the first exercise session. This should then be followed by centralisation of pain. Once the pain no longer spreads outwards and is felt in the midline only, the intensity of the pain will decrease rapidly over a period of two to three days and in another three days the pain should disappear entirely.

If, following an initial pain increase, the pain continues to increase in intensity or spreads to places further away from the spine, you should stop exercising and seek advice. In other words, do not continue with any of the exercises if your symptoms are much worse immediately after exercising and remain worse the next day; or if, during exercising, symptoms are produced or increased in the arm below the elbow.

As discussed earlier, once you have started this exercise programme, you should expect *new* pains to develop. These are different from your original pain and are usually felt in areas of the neck and shoulder girdle, which were previously not affected. New pains are the result of performing movements your body is not used

As long as your pain is slowly improving, continue with the exercises that have led to this improvement. Do not change anything in your established routine. It may be tempting to add other exercises, but this may disrupt your progress. Wait until improvement stops before considering any other activity or exercise.

to and, provided you continue with the exercises, they will wear off in three to four days.

If your symptoms have been present rather continuously for many weeks or months, you should not expect to be pain-free in two to three days. The response will be slower, but, if you are doing the correct exercises, it will only be a matter of time before the pain subsides.

Starting the exercise programme

When you commence this exercise programme you should stop any other exercises that you may have been shown elsewhere or happen to do regularly – for example, for fitness or sport. If you want to continue with exercises other than the ones described in this book for neck problems, you should wait until your pains have subsided completely.

It is recommended that you adopt the sitting position when learning to perform the exercises. Once you fully master them you may exercise in sitting or standing, whichever is most suitable.

However, if the pain is too severe to tolerate the exercises in sitting, it may be necessary to commence exercising while lying down. In the lying position the pain will be reduced, because the head and neck are better supported and the compressive forces on the spine are considerably less than in sitting. If you are sixty years of age or older, it is also advisable to commence exercising while lying down. People of older age groups occasionally experience dizziness or light-headedness when performing extension exercises with the head. If these symptoms should persist, you must stop the exercises and seek advice. On the other hand, when the initial attempts at extension exercises in lying do not have any ill effects, you can safely proceed to exercising in sitting.

If, due to medical problems, it is difficult or not advisable for you to lie flat, you should restrict yourself to exercising in the upright sitting position.

Overview

In order to treat **present** neck problems successfully you must do the following:

- *at all times:* correct your posture and maintain the correct posture
- *when in acute pain:* if possible, perform Exercises 1 and 2; if not possible, then do Exercises 3 and 4
- *when pain is more to one side and not responding:* first Exercise 5, later Exercises 1 and 2
- *when acute pain has subsided:* Exercises 6 and 7, always followed by Exercises 1 and 2.

In order to **prevent** future neck problems successfully you must do the following:

- *at all times:* maintain good postural habits
- *when no pain or stiffness:* Exercise 6 two times per day, *always* followed by Exercises 1 and 2
- *at first sign of recurrence:* postural correction and Exercises 1 and 2 at regular intervals – that is, ten times per session and six to eight sessions per day.

IT IS STRONGLY RECOMMENDED THAT YOU FAMILIARISE YOURSELF WITH **ALL** THE EXERCISES AND INFORMATION IN CHAPTERS 5 AND 6.

Exercise 1: Head retraction in sitting

Head retraction means pulling the head backwards.

- sit on a chair or stool, look straight ahead and allow yourself to relax completely Your head will protrude a little as you do this (Photo 32). Now you are ready to start the first and most important exercise.

- move your head slowly but steadily backwards until it is pulled back as far as you can manage (Photo 33). It is important to keep your chin tucked down and in as you do this. In other words, you must remain looking straight ahead and should not tilt the head backwards as in looking up. When your head is pulled back as far as possible, you have assumed the retracted head posture (Photo 33).

- once you have maintained this position for a few seconds, you should relax and automatically your head and neck will protrude again (Photo 32)

- each time you repeat this movement cycle you must make sure that the backward movement of head and neck is performed to the maximum possible degree

- the exercise can be made more effective by adding overpressure. This is done by placing both hands on the chin and firmly pushing the head back even further (Photo 34).

This exercise is used mainly in the treatment of neck pain.

When used in the *treatment* of neck pain, the exercise should be repeated ten times per session and the sessions should be spread evenly six to eight times throughout the day until you go to bed at night. This means that you should repeat the sessions about every two hours. When used in the *prevention* of neck pain, the exercise should be repeated five or six times as often as required.

Should you experience severe pain on attempting this exercise, you must replace it with *Exercise 3: Head retraction in lying*.

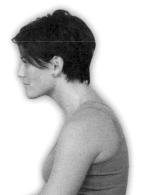
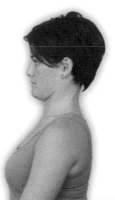
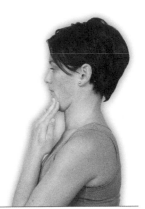

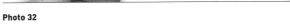

Photo 32   **Photo 33**   **Photo 34**

Exercise 2: Neck extension in sitting

Extension means bending backwards. This exercise should always follow Exercise 1.

- remain seated, repeat Exercise 1 a few times, and then hold your head in the retracted position (Photo 35). Now you are ready to start Exercise 2.

- lift your chin up and tilt your head backwards as in looking up at the sky (Photo 36). Do not allow your neck to move forwards as you do this.

- with your head tilted back as far as possible, you must rotate your head from side to side so that your nose moves just half an inch (about 2 cm) to the right and then to the left of the midline (Photos 37 and 38), all the time attempting to move head and neck even further backwards. This movement should be repeated quite rhythmically and not too slowly.

- once you have done this for a few seconds, you should return your head to the starting position. Again, each time you repeat this movement cycle you must make sure that neck extension is performed to the maximum possible degree.

This exercise can be used both in the treatment and in the prevention of neck pain.

Exercise 2 is to be performed ten times per session and the sessions should be spread evenly six to eight times per day until you go to bed. If your pain is too severe to tolerate Exercise 2, you should replace it with *Exercise 3: Head retraction in lying*.

Once you are fully practised in Exercises 1 and 2 separately, you can combine these two exercises successfully into one exercise.

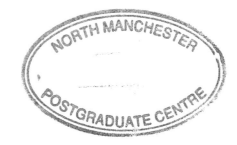
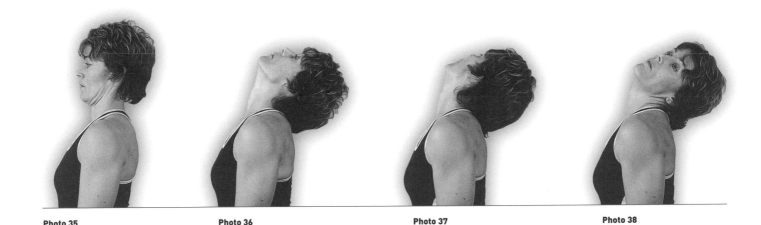

Photo 35   Photo 36   Photo 37   Photo 38

Exercise 3: Head retraction in lying

- lie face up with your head at a free-standing edge of the bed – for example, lie across a double bed or with your head at the foot-end of a single bed. Rest your head and shoulders flat on the bed and do not use a pillow (Photo 39). Now you are ready to start Exercise 3.
- push the back of your head into the mattress and at the same time pull your chin in (Photo 40). The overall effect should be that your head and neck move backwards as far as possible while you keep facing the ceiling.
- once you have maintained this position for a few seconds, you should relax and automatically the head and neck return to the starting position (Photo 39). Each time you repeat this movement cycle, you should make sure that the backward movement of head and neck is carried out to the maximum possible degree.

This exercise is used mainly in the treatment of severe neck pain.

When you have completed ten head retractions, you must evaluate the effects of this exercise on the pain. If the pain has centralised or decreased in intensity, you can safely continue this procedure. In this case you should repeat the exercise ten times per session and spread the sessions evenly six to eight times throughout the day or night. However, if the pain has increased considerably or extends further away from the spine, or if you have developed pins and needles or numbness in the fingers, then you must stop the exercise and seek advice.

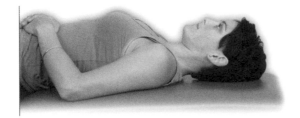

Photo 39

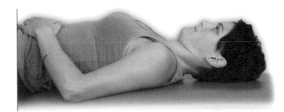

Photo 40

Exercise 4: Neck extension in lying

This exercise should always follow Exercise 3. Again, you must lie face up on the bed.

- before you can start Exercise 4 you must place one hand under your head and move up along the bed until the head, neck and the top of your shoulders are extended over the edge of the bed (Photo 41)

- while supporting your head with one hand you should lower it slowly down towards the floor (Photo 42)

- now remove your hand (Photo 43), tilt your head and neck as far backwards as you can and try to see as much as possible of the floor directly under you

- in this position you must repeatedly rotate your head from side to side so that your nose moves just half an inch (about 2 cm) to the right and then to the left of the midline (Photo 44), attempting to move your head and neck further backwards as you do this. This movement should be repeated quite rhythmically and not too slowly.

- once you have reached the maximum amount of extension, you should try to relax in this position for about thirty seconds

- in order to return to the resting position, you must first place one hand behind your head, then assist your head back to the horizontal position and move down along the bed until your head is lying on the bed again.

Following this exercise, it is important that you *do not* rise immediately but rest for a few minutes with your head flat on the bed. Do not use a pillow.

As Exercise 3, this exercise is used mainly in the treatment of severe neck pain.

Until the acute symptoms have subsided, Exercise 4 is to follow Exercise 3 and should be done only once per session. Once you no longer have severe pain, Exercises 3 and 4 should be replaced with Exercises 1 and 2. By now you will have noticed that, except for the position in which they are performed, Exercises 3 and 4 are really the same as Exercises 1 and 2.

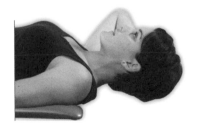

Photo 41

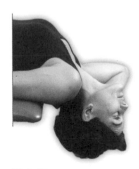

Photo 42

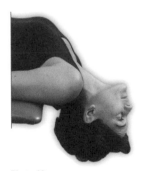

Photo 43

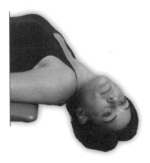

Photo 44

Exercise 5: Sidebending of the neck

- sit on a chair, repeat Exercise 1 a few times, and then hold your head in the retracted position (Photo 45). Now you are ready to start Exercise 5.

- bend your neck sideways and move your head towards the side on which you feel most of the pain (Photo 46). Do not allow the head to turn so that your nose moves towards your shoulder; in other words, you should keep looking straight ahead and bring your ear towards your shoulder. It is important that you keep the head well retracted as you do this.

- the exercise can be made more effective by placing the hand of your most painful side over the top of your head and gently but firmly pulling your head even further towards the painful side (Photo 47)

- once you have maintained this position for a few seconds, you should return the head to the starting position.

This exercise is used specifically for the treatment of pain felt only to one side of the neck that does not improve with Exercises 1 and 2, or for the treatment of pain felt much more to the one side than to the other.

Until the symptoms have centralised, Exercise 5 is to be repeated ten times per session and the sessions are to be spread evenly six to eight times throughout the day.

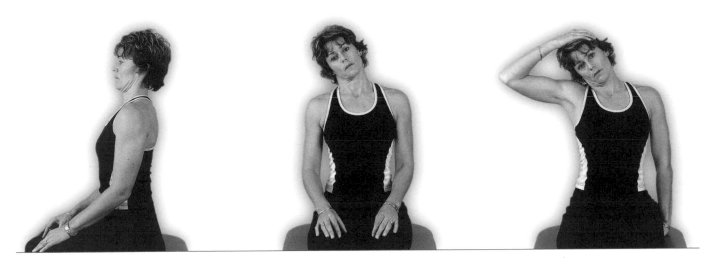

Photo 45

Photo 46

Photo 47

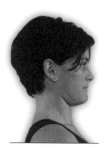

Photo 48

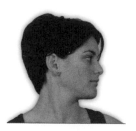

Photo 49

Exercise 6: Neck rotation

Rotation means turning to the right and left.

- sit on a chair, repeat Exercise 1 a few times, and then hold your head in the retracted position (Photo 48). Now you are ready to start Exercise 6.

- while still retracted, turn your head far to the right and then far to the left (Photo 49). It is important that you keep the head well retracted as you do this. If you experience more pain on turning to the one side than to the other, you should continue to exercise by rotating to the **most painful** side; on repetition the pain should gradually centralise or decrease in intensity. However, should the pain increase and fail to centralise, you must continue to exercise by rotating to the **least painful** side. Once you have the same amount of pain or no pain and only stiffness when turning to either side, you should continue to exercise by rotating to both sides.

- the exercise can be made more effective by using both hands and gently but firmly pushing your head even further into rotation (Photos 50, 51 and 52)

- once you have maintained the position of maximum rotation for a few seconds, you should return your head to the starting position.

This exercise can be used in the treatment as well as the prevention of neck pain.

When used in the treatment of pain or stiffness of the neck, the exercise is to be performed ten times per session and the sessions are to be spread evenly six to eight times throughout the day. Whether centralisation or reduction of the pain has taken place or not, Exercise 6 must always be followed by Exercises 1 and 2. When used in the prevention of neck problems, the exercise should be repeated five or six times every once in a while or as often as required (for example, when stiffness is first felt).

Note that in the majority of cases, stiffness on rotation is caused by a blockage at the back of the joint that must be dealt with by performing Exercises 1 and 2. Only do Exercise 6 if your neck pain or headache is not helped by Exercises 1 and 2.

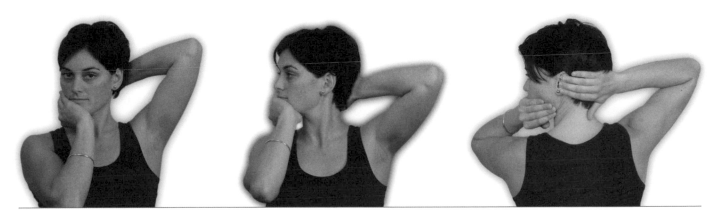

Photo 50   **Photo 51**   **Photo 52**

Exercise 7: Neck flexion in sitting

Flexion means bending forwards.

- sit on a chair, look straight ahead and allow yourself to relax completely (Photo 53). Now you are ready to start Exercise 7.

- drop your head forwards and let it rest with the chin as close as possible to the chest (Photo 54)

- place your hands behind the back of your head and interlock your fingers. Let your arms relax so that the elbows point down towards the floor. In this position the weight of the arms will pull your head down further and bring your chin closer to the chest (Photo 55).

- the exercise can be made more effective by using your hands to gently but firmly pull your head onto your chest

- once you have maintained the position of maximum neck flexion for a few seconds, you should return your head to the starting position

This exercise is used specifically for the treatment of headaches, but can also be applied to resolve residual neck pain or stiffness once the acute symptoms have subsided.

In both cases it should be repeated only two or three times per session and the sessions should be spread evenly six to eight times throughout the day. When used in the treatment of headaches, Exercise 7 should be performed in conjunction with Exercise 1. When used in the treatment of neck pain or stiffness, Exercise 7 must *always* be followed by Exercises 1 and 2.

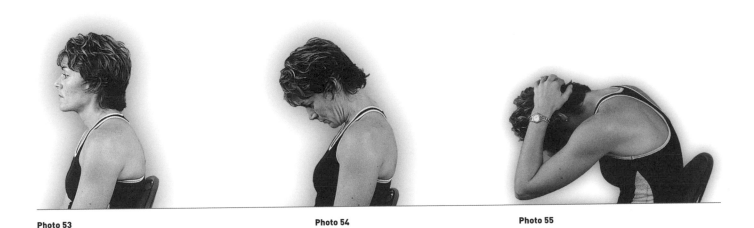

Photo 53   **Photo 54**   **Photo 55**

When to apply the exercises

Chapter six

When you are in significant pain

If the pain is very severe, you may be able to get out of bed with difficulty, but certain movements will be impossible and often you cannot find a comfortable position in which to sit or work. Even though you have severe pain, you should always attempt to commence with *Exercise 1: Head retraction in sitting* (Photo 56). Many people find that this exercise gives substantial relief from pain, and they do not have to start exercising in lying. As soon as possible, even on the first day, you should add *Exercise 2: Neck extension in sitting* (Photo 57). You should continue the above exercises until you feel considerably better. Once you no longer have acute pain, you should follow the exercise programme as outlined for when acute pain has subsided.

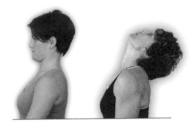

Photo 56
Exercise 1

Photo 57
Exercise 2

If you have performed three or four sessions of Exercise 1 spread over a period of fifteen minutes and the pain remains too severe to tolerate this exercise, you should stop and replace it with *Exercise 3: Head retraction in lying* (Photo 58). Your symptoms should gradually reduce and centralise so that there is some improvement by the time you have completed a few sessions. *Exercise 4: Neck extension in lying* (Photo 59) should be added as soon as you have become well practised in Exercise 3

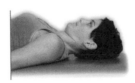

Photo 58
Exercise 3

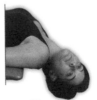

Photo 59
Exercise 4

and your symptoms have improved to some extent, or when you cease to improve with Exercise 3. Introducing Exercise 4 varies from person to person, but the sooner you can do this the better. It is important that you carefully watch the pain pattern. You are exercising correctly if in a few days the pain moves towards the base or the centre of the neck and decreases in intensity. In the end the pain should disappear entirely and be replaced by a feeling of strain or stiffness.

When you have improved significantly – usually two to three days after you commence the exercises in lying, possibly earlier – you may gradually reduce the number of sessions of Exercises 3 and 4, and as you do this you should introduce and gradually increase Exercises 1 and 2. In another few days you are only performing exercises in sitting and you will find that they give the same pain relief as you previously obtained by exercising in lying. At this stage the periods of time that you are completely free of pain are becoming more frequent and start to last longer.

Again, once you feel considerably better and no longer have acute pain, you should continue the exercise programme as outlined for when acute pain has subsided.

When you have headaches

Headaches can often be relieved by some of the recommended exercises, usually Exercises 1 and 7. It will not do any harm to perform these exercises for a couple of days in order to find out whether you benefit from them or not.

The first three days you should perform *Exercise 1: Head retraction in sitting* (Photo 60) at regular intervals and whenever you feel a headache is developing. If this reduces your headaches but does not abolish them completely, you should add *Exercise 7: Neck flexion in sitting* (Photo 61). In particular the headaches that spread over the top of your head to above or behind the eyes are often relieved with this exercise. You may even be able to prevent the development of such headaches by performing this exercise as soon as you feel minor strain building up.

In case your headaches are not relieved by these two exercises, try sustaining the end range position of Exercise 1 by adding overpressure (see page 42) for 1-2 minutes (Photo 62).

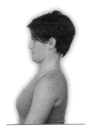 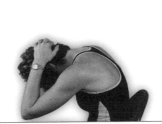 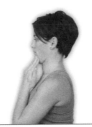

Photo 60
Exercise 1

Photo 61
Exercise 7

Photo 62
Adding overpressure

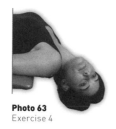

Photo 63
Exercise 4

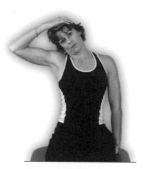

Photo 64
Exercise 5

**Exercise 5 must always be
followed by Exercises 1 and 2**

You should also for the next three days do *Exercise 4: Neck extension in lying* (Photo 63) followed by Exercises 1 and 2 and postural correction. As your symptoms are improving you may gradually stop Exercise 4, but you must continue with the other two exercises.

If you are unable to influence your headaches with any of the exercises or if your headaches become much worse during exercising and remain worse over the next day, you should stop exercising and seek advice.

No response or benefit

When pain is felt only to one side of the spine or much more to the one side than to the other, the exercises recommended so far sometimes fail to bring relief. If this is the case, you should commence with *Exercise 5: Sidebending of the neck* (Photo 64). Whether centralisation or reduction of the pain has taken place or not, Exercise 5 must always be followed by Exercises 1 and 2. After two or three days of practise you may notice that the pain is distributed more evenly across the cervical spine or has centralised. Now you may gradually reduce Exercise 5.

When you are considerably better and the pain has fully centralised, you should continue with the exercise programme as outlined for when acute pain has subsided.

When acute pain has subsided

Once the acute pain has passed, you may still feel some pain or stiffness when moving in certain ways. You will notice this most when turning your head to one side or the other or tilting your head and neck forwards to look down. It is likely that at this stage healing of overstretched or damaged soft tissues has taken place. Now you must ensure that the elasticity of these soft tissues and the flexibility of your spine as a whole are restored without causing further damage.

If you have pain on turning the head to the right or the left, you should practise *Exercise 6: Neck rotation* (Photo 65), and if you have pain on bending the head forwards, you need to practise *Exercise 7: Neck flexion in sitting* (Photo 66). Each time you repeat the exercise you must move to the edge of the pain and then release the pressure. The pain should disappear entirely over a period of two to three weeks. Each session of Exercises 6 and 7 should always be concluded with a few repetitions of Exercises 1 and 2.

If you feel stiffness only on these movements, you should do the same exercises but apply overpressure with your hands at the end of each movement. By exercising in this way you achieve movement to the maximum possible degree. In a period of three to six weeks you should have restored normal function.

Once you are completely symptom free, you should follow the guidelines given to prevent recurrence of neck problems. Continue with the exercise programme as outlined for when you have no pain or stiffness.

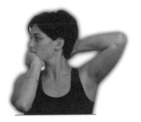

Photo 65
Exercise 6

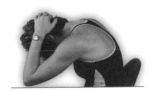

Photo 66
Exercise 7

When you have no pain or stiffness

Many people with neck problems have lengthy spells in which they experience little or no pain. If in the past or recently you have had one or more episodes of neck pain, you should start the exercise programme even though you may be pain-free at the moment. However, in this situation it is not necessary to do all the exercises or to exercise every two hours.

To prevent recurrence of neck problems you should perform *Exercise 6: Neck rotation* (Photo 67) followed by *Exercises 1* and *2: Head retraction in sitting* and *Neck extension in sitting* (Photo 68 and 69) on a regular basis, preferably in the morning and at night. Furthermore, whenever you feel minor strain developing during work or while sitting, you should perform Exercises 1 and 2. It is even more important that you watch your posture at all times and never again let postural stresses be the cause of neck pain. These exercises will have very little or no effect if you constantly

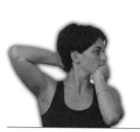
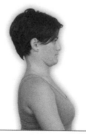
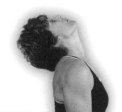

Photo 67
Exercise 6

Photo 68
Exercise 1

Photo 69
Exercise 2

fall back into poor posture. While it may be necessary to exercise in the manner described above for the rest of your life, it is absolutely essential that you develop and maintain good postural habits.

As it takes only one minute to perform one session of Exercise 6 and another minute to combine Exercises 1 and 2 and repeat them ten times, lack of time should never be used as an excuse for not being able to do these exercises.

Recurrence

At the first sign of recurrence of neck pain you should immediately perform *Exercises 1* and *2: Head retraction in sitting* and *Neck extension in sitting*. If your pain is already too severe to tolerate these exercises or if they fail to reduce the pain, you must quickly introduce *Exercises 3* and *4: Head retraction in lying* and *Neck extension in lying*. If you have one-sided symptoms that do not centralise with any of these exercises, you should start with *Exercise 5: Sidebending of the neck*. Again, you must pay extra attention to your posture, regularly perform postural correction and maintain the correct posture as much as you can.

- maintenance of good posture is essential. You are unable to maintain a cervical lordosis if you sit or stand incorrectly.
- keep your head up at all times. When you allow the head to droop as in reading, knitting, sewing and performing desk tasks, you place further strains on the already overstretched or injured tissues.
- do not roll the head around and avoid quick movements, especially turning the head quickly
- avoid those positions and movements that initially caused your problems. You must allow some time for healing to take place.
- do not sleep with more pillows than necessary. If you are comfortable with one pillow, then use only one. The contents of the pillow should be adjustable in order to provide proper support for the neck.
- when you remain uncomfortable at night, you may benefit from a cervical roll
- do not sleep face down, as this places great strains on the neck
- do not lie in the bath for long times, as this bends your head and neck forwards, excessively
- carefully start with the self-treatment exercises. Remember, an initial pain increase can be expected when commencing any of the exercises. This pain should reduce or centralise as you repeat the movements.

The McKenzie Institute International

 If you wish to find out more about Robin McKenzie, the McKenzie Method, the McKenzie Institute International or if you would like to locate a credentialled or diplomaed member or associate of the McKenzie Institute, visit www.mckenziemdt.org, call the McKenzie Institute International Head Office in New Zealand on +64 4 299-6645 or refer to the list below for the branch nearest you:

Head Office (NZ)	www.mckenziemdt.org	Hungary	www.mckenziemodszer.hu
Argentina	www.mckenziemdt.com.ar	Italy	www.mckenzie-italia.com
Australia	www.backcare4u.com.au	Japan	www.mckenziemdt.org
Austria	www.mckenziemdt.org	New Zealand	www.mckenziemdt.org.nz
Benelux	www.mckenzie.nl	Nigeria	www.mckenziemdt.org
Brazil	www.mckenzie.org.br	Norway	www.mckenziemdt.org
Canada	www.mckenzieinstitute.ca	Poland	www.mckenzie.pl
Croatia	www.mckenziemdt.org	Saudi Arabia	www.mckenziemdt.org
Czech Republic	www.mckenzie.cz	Slovakia	www.mckenzie.cz
Denmark	www.mckenzie.dk	Slovenia	www.mg-mg.si/McK/
Finland	www.suomenmckenzieinstituutti.fi	Sweden	www.mckenzie.a.se
France	www.mckenziemdt.org	Switzerland	www.mckenziemdt.org
Germany	www.mckenzie.de	USA	www.mckenziemdt.org
Hellas/Cyprus	www.mckenziehellas.gr	United Kingdom	www.mckenzieinstitute.co.uk

The Original McKenzie® lumbar rolls described in this book are available worldwide from the following licensed distributors, as is *Treat Your Own Back*, the companion volume to this book, by the same author.

Head Office and New Zealand
Spinal Publications New Zealand Ltd
PO Box 2026, Raumati Beach, New Zealand
Phone: +64 4 299-7020
www.spinalpublications.co.nz

Argentina	www.physicaltherapydistributors.com	Italy	www.spinalpublications.it
Australia	www.backcare4u.com.au	Japan	http://www5.ocn.ne.jp/~ped
Belgium	www.ergoaktiv.be	Mexico	Email: tfsirs@yahoo.com.mx
Brazil	www.mckenzie.br.org	Netherlands	www.bodybow.nl
Czech Rep. (books)	www.mckenzie.cz	North America	www.optp.com
Czech Rep. (rolls)	www.backcare.xf.cz	Scandinavia	www.scanergo.se
Germany	www.mckenzie-shop.de	Southern Africa	www.bacline.com
Hong Kong	Email: bhltd@netvigator.com	United Kingdom	www.mobilisrolyan.com
India	Email: medtechi@gmail.com	Western Europe (various countries)	www.ergonline.eu
Israel	www.teamcarempt.com/israel		

For the most up to date list of distributors, visit www.spinalpublications.co.nz